Emergen

M000199792

Eye and Orbit

Senior Editor:
Dietrich Jehle, MD, FACEP, RDMS
Professor of Emergency Medicine
Director of Emergency Ultrasonography
University at Buffalo School of Medicine
Buffalo, New York

Authors:
Sean Bouvet, MD, RDMS
Ultrasound Fellow, Department of Emergency Medicine
University at Buffalo, Buffalo, New York
Clinical Instructor of Emergency Medicine
Johns Hopkins School of Medicine, Baltimore, MD

Beau Braden, DO
Department of Emergency Medicine
University at Buffalo, Buffalo, New York

Marcus Hendry, MD
Department of Emergency Medicine
University at Buffalo, Buffalo, New York

John Nagel, MD
Department of Emergency Medicine
University at Buffalo, Buffalo, New York

James Reidy, MD
Associate Professor of Ophthalmology
Director, Cornea Service
University at Buffalo School of Medicine
Buffalo, New York

Acknowledgments

We would like to thank the many emergency physicians and ophthalmologists that have pioneered the use of bedside ophthalmic ultrasound as a diagnostic tool. It has forever changed the way we practice medicine. In addition, we would like to thank those that have published research that supports our ability to use this tool with confidence. Special thanks go to those that have taught us these techniques and fostered our interest in such a valuable imaging modality. To them we express our gratitude and acknowledge an everlasting debt.

Several individuals who deserve particular recognition for their invaluable contributions are Fritz Sticht and Dr. Mark Comaratta. Fritz deserves special recognition for the work he did as an imaging specialist and medical illustrator to bring this text to press. Dr. Comaratta is an ophthalmologist who specializes in retina pathology. He provided us with a large number of the ultrasound images that we incorporated into this text. We would also like to thank Drs. Fernando Lopez, Michael Blaivas, James Rippey, Donna D'Souza and Reiner Van Tonder who provided additional ultrasound images for this text. There are many physicians who provided constructive feedback on early versions of this text as members of the Ultrasound Track of the Emergency Medicine Residency at the State University of New York at Buffalo, and to them we are deeply indebted.

Finally, we would like to thank our families for their continuing support of all that we do. The support, patience and understanding of our spouses and children are truly valued and deeply appreciated.

Legal Notice

The authors of this book have attempted to ensure that all information contained within is accurate and current with respect to generally accepted practices at the time of publication. However, neither the author nor publisher of this book claims that all information contained herein is wholly accurate and complete. They disclaim responsibility for errors, omissions, and for results and consequences of the use of the information within the book. They encourage the confirmation of this information with other resources. This work is copyrighted under United States copyright law.

Preface

Emergency Ultrasound of the Eye and Orbit was written and published to provide a basic reference to emergency physicians and ophthalmologists. While the intended audience includes emergency physicians who already are using bedside ultrasonography for the evaluation of their patients, this book includes the basics of physics and instrumentation, scanning techniques, and effects and artifacts that apply to other uses beyond ophthalmic ultrasound. This book will focus on grey scale applications of ophthalmic ultrasound that can easily be learned by those performing other non-ophthalmologic grey scale studies.

A growing body of literature supports the use of ultrasound by practitioners to diagnose a variety of significant eye pathologies. This book emphasizes the use of ultrasound to evaluate emergent and urgent ophthalmologic conditions. While some chronic or non-urgent findings will be discussed, these are generally addressed in the context of differentiating these from more emergent conditions. Clearly, there are a number of vision-threatening conditions for which ultrasonography can help the physician secure the appropriate and timely treatment.

We submit this book as both a teaching tool and a bedside reference for emergency ophthalmic ultrasound.

TABLE OF CONTENTS

INTRODUCTION

Many patients come to the emergency department with complaints of visual change or loss, ocular trauma, eye pain or other conditions which necessitate an accurate assessment of the eye and/or orbit. A number of techniques are available to aid the physician – direct ophthalmoscopy, slit-lamp examination, and tonometry, to name a few.

There are numerous times, however, when these modalities are insufficient or impractical for use by the physician evaluating the eye. Cataracts in the lens, vitreous opacities or a large hyphema may make it impossible to perform a complete evaluation of the posterior globe by direct ophthalmoscopy alone. Trauma to the region of the eye may produce such significant swelling of the eyelids and periorbital tissues that it becomes difficult to even separate the lids and assess for pupillary response, let alone other conditions. When the direct clinical evaluation of the eye is compromised by such conditions, ultrasound may offer a fast, non-invasive modality to study the eye and determine the need for ophthalmologic intervention. Ultrasound also offers a way to assess and record information about the eye not previously possible with older modalities.

Ultrasound has been used by ophthalmologists for several decades. In the late 1950's, A-scan ultrasound was used to evaluate intraocular tumors. By the mid-1970's, B-scan equipment was commercially available to ophthalmologists, albeit using probes exclusively designed for ophthalmologic applications. As multi-purpose high frequency probes are now available for many of the portable ultrasound machines found in emergency departments, emergency physicians can now take advantage of these diagnostic capabilities.

With the correct equipment and some practice, the emergency physician and ophthalmologist can learn to assess causes of acute non-traumatic visual loss, such as vitreous hemorrhage, vitreous detachment, and retinal detachment. Traumatic problems can also be evaluated, including foreign body penetration and lens subluxation or dislocation. Structures posterior to the eye can be imaged as well. Knowing the normal appearance of these structures and the changes corresponding to various conditions can help the physician identify orbital cellulitis or increased intracranial pressure.

Although, the central retinal artery and vein can be imaged with color Doppler equipment, the application of this is beyond the scope of this basic book. Color Doppler imaging will only be briefly addressed as it is covered in detail in several comprehensive ophthalmic ultrasound texts.

SECTION 1: PHYSICS

Introduction

More so than most imaging modalities, ultrasonography is highly operator dependent, and interpretation of images is best when done in a fluid rather than static manner. The physician performing the exam must therefore have a solid understanding of the basic principles of ultrasound physics in order to assure that the images obtained are of sufficient quality, and that these images are interpreted correctly. The following discussion provides an overview of principles that should be understood in order to obtain quality bedside studies.

Sound Waves

Sound by definition is radiant mechanical energy transmitted in longitudinal pressure waves within a given medium. The characteristics of sound are those that apply to wave theory in general, in that they are measured in terms of frequency/period, wavelength, and amplitude. Discussion of ultrasound requires an understanding of these terms.

•**Frequency** is defined as the number of disturbances, or pressure waves, in a given time period. The standard measurement is number per second, symbolized by Hertz (Hz). The standard human hearing range is approximately 20 Hz to 20 kHz, with anything over 20 kHz referred to as ultrasound. Standard medical diagnostic ultrasonography uses frequency in the 2-10 MHz, and up to 60 MHz in specific diagnostics. Given that the length of the average eye is approximately 24 mm, the ophthalmologic ultrasound exam does not require much tissue penetration. High frequency probes, with frequencies of 7.5-15 MHz, are generally utilized in the emergency department, which provide better tissue resolution. There are also a number of very high-resolution ophthalmic probes now available to the practicing ophthalmologist that use much higher frequencies (20 – 60 MHz) for specialized diagnostic evaluation of the anterior chamber.

•**Wavelength** is the distance between corresponding points on consecutive waves. This is a function of frequency and the speed of sound in the particular medium in which it is traveling. It is the wavelength that determines the axial spatial resolution one can achieve with diagnostic ultrasound. The shorter the wavelength is (i.e. higher frequency), the greater detail or resolution can be achieved; however, the maximum depth of penetration is shallower.

•**Amplitude** is a measure from peak to trough of a given wave, which represents the intensity, or power, of the sound.

Properties of Diagnostic Ultrasound Waves

All sound waves, including those used in ultrasonography, display certain physical principles. Among these are reflection, refraction, absorption, and interference. In human tissue, these characteristics are manifested as follows.

• Diagnostic ultrasound depends on the reflection of echoed waves back to the transducer from which they originate. In order for these waves to be measured, they must be reflected by an interface that is perpendicular to the direction of the wave. Any waves that strike an interface at an **angle of incidence** that is not perpendicular will be either refracted or reflected in a direction that results in lower measured amplitude by the transducer.

• If the ultrasound wave travels into a significantly denser medium, there is greater **absorption, reflection** and scatter of the ultrasound wave.

• The **velocity** of the ultrasound wave varies with the density of the tissue. Sound travels faster in solids than liquids; and faster in liquids than gas. The speed of sound in the vitreous of the eye is approximately 1,532 m/sec and 1,641 m/sec in the lens.

• **Acoustic impedance** is a function of the velocity of sound in the tissue and the density of the tissue. The greater the difference in **impedance** between two tissues creating an interface, the better able one is to distinguish between the two. For example, the difference in impedance between the lens and anterior chamber and that between the retina and vitreous chamber allows for a strong reflection. (Figure 1-1 A&B)

• **Refraction** is the bending of the sound beam that

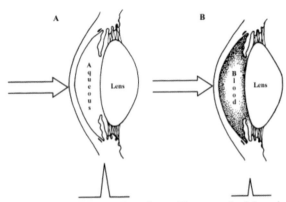

Figure 1-1 A&B Acoustic Impedance. The strength of the echo produced at the interface between two tissues is dependent on the acoustic impedance which is related to tissue density. The greater the difference in impedance between neighboring structures, the stronger the returning echoes. Thus the echo produced from the interface between aqueous and the anterior lens capsule (A) is greater than that produced by the interface between hemorrhage and the anterior lens capsule (B). Reprinted with permission from Byrne S, Green R. Ultrasound of the Eye and Orbit, 2nd ed. Philadelphia, PA: Mosby; 2002.

occurs at an interface between two medium that transmit sound at different speeds.

• A final concept is **attenuation**, which is the decrease in amplitude that occurs over a given distance. Attenuation is what limits the depth at which ultrasound can be used to visualize structures. Higher attenuation occurs with higher frequency. Thus higher frequencies provide greater resolution and are used to look at more superficial structures (eye/orbit and vessels), while lower frequencies provide lower resolution yet allow visualization of deeper structures (abdominal ultrasound).

Image Production

• The raw data that is collected from echoed ultrasound waves can be represented by a series of spikes graphed over time, which given a relatively constant speed of sound transmission, corresponds to distance from the transducer. This representation is also known as "**A-mode**" ultrasound. (Figure 1-2)

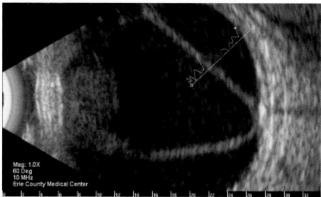

Figure 1-2 A and B-Mode. This image of a retinal detachment demonstrates the appearance of sound waves transmitted and returned to a transducer in both A-mode (one dimensional spikes) and B-mode (2D image).

• When this data is used by the computer to generate a 2-dimensional image, this is termed "**B-mode**" ultrasound. A-mode scanning has a well described

benefit in ophthalmic scanning and a thorough ultra-
sonographic exam of the eye includes the combination of A and B-mode techniques. For the purpose
of emergency scans, however, B-mode information
alone is generally adequate. As in other applications
of emergency bedside ultrasound, the purpose of the
focused exam is usually to answer a specific ques-
tion, such as "Is there a membranous detachment?"
This can easily be answered with B-mode imaging.
The width and the peak on the A-mode scan are occasionally necessary to provide quantitative information to help distinguish a posterior vitreous detachment from a retinal detachment. (Figure 1-3)

• **Orientation** to the monitor is standardized so that
objects nearer to the transducer (termed the **near
field**) are towards the top of the screen (to the left
with opthamology equipment), and those farther
(termed the **far field**) are at the bottom with an
emergency medicine small parts probe. The **focal
zone** is the middle of the viewing field. One should
try to position the structure of interest within the
focal zone as the lateral resolution is greatest here.
The left of the screen is the direction of the probe
marker when using an emergency medicine small
parts probe and the top of the screen with traditional
ophthalmic ultrasound equipment. (Figure 1-4)

• Structures are described in terms of the amount of
echoes they generate, or their **echogenicity**. They
are described in terms relative to the tissues around
them. Hypoechoic structures produce less reflection

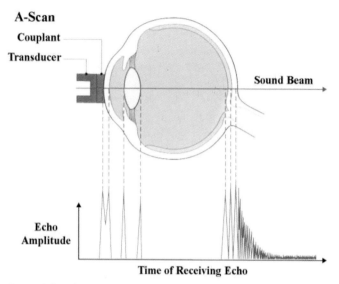

Figure 1-3 Width and Peak on a Normal A-mode Scan. Information from the A-mode scanning is occasionally helpful to provide quantitative information that can help distinguish a posterior vitreous detachment from a retinal detachment. A posterior vitreous detachment is thinner and less echogenic than the retinal detachment, and thus it has a smaller and narrower spike on A-mode imaging. Reprinted with permission from Spalton D, Hitchings R, Hunter P. Atlas of clinical ophthalmology, 3rd ed. Philadelphia, PA: Mosby; 2005.

than the surrounding tissue and will appear darker on the monitor. Isoechoic structures have similar echogenicity compared with surrounding tissue, making distinction between different tissues more difficult. Finally, hyperechoic structures have a relatively higher echogenicity and will appear brighter on the monitor. Gaseous structures do not allow

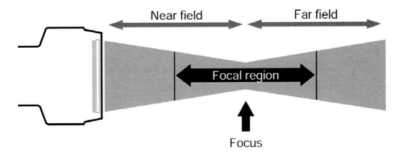

Figure 1-4 Focal Zone. The best resolution is obtained when the region of greatest interest is in the focal zone of the transducer. This focal zone is the area between the near and far field of the probe.

adequate US transmission and can interfere with imaging. Silicone oil, used in some types of retinal surgery, blocks ultrasound waves. Bone, because of its density, reflects most US waves and prohibits visualization of deeper structures. Fluid is relatively hypoechoic in comparison to soft tissue structures. In ophthalmic scanning, echogenic structures at the posterior pole of the globe can be well visualized within the hypoechoic vitreous. (Figure 1-5 A-C)

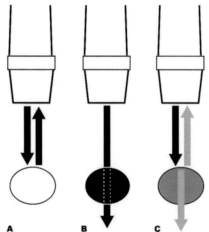

*Figure 1-5 A-C Sonographic Appearances.
A) Echogenic image, where the structure
reflects most sound waves. The structure
is echogenic or white on the screen. B)
Anechoic image, where most of the sound
waves are transmitted through a homogeneous structure. The structure is anechoic or
dark on the screen. Most anechoic structures
are cystic; however, they may be a solid or
soft tissue density. The posterior echoes can
usually help define the dark structure: cystic
structures result in posterior enhancement;
soft tissue or solid structures have no posterior enhancement. C) Imaging of a structure
of mixed tissue density that both transmits
and reflects ultrasound waves. The structure
appears gray on the screen.*

SECTION 2: INSTRUMENTATION

Transducers

An ultrasound transducer is the device that converts electrical impulses generated by the machine transmitter into mechanical (acoustic) energy. Transducers also then convert echoed acoustic energy back into electrical impulses that are interpreted by the machine. This process is accomplished by means of vibration of piezoelectric crystals within the transducer. Various configurations of crystals within a probe can be used to obtain images that best suit the need of the particular exam. Behind the crystals, all probes have a layer of dampening material that limits vibration, shortens pulses, and improves resolution. (Figure 2-1 A&B)

Mechanical transducers have a single element that either oscillates or spins within the transducer head. **Electronic** transducers which are more commonly used in practice today contain a number of crystals that are arranged in an array. The type of array dictates what type of image is produced. The area of the transducer head which contacts the imaged surface is called the footprint. Various arrays and footprints are best suited to particular applications.

• **Linear array** transducers have crystals arranged in a linear fashion within a flat transducer head. This produces a rectangular image equal in width to that of the transducer head. These are commonly used with higher frequencies and are best

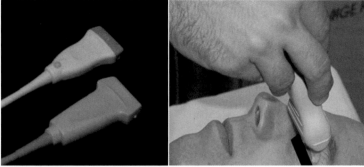

Figure 2-1 A&B Transducers Utilized in the Emergency Department. Most emergency physicians will utilize a small parts probe (A) when doing ophthalmic imaging in the emergency department. This small parts probe can also be utilized for vascular access, DVT studies and the evaluation of superficial masses. The probe and gel are placed gently over the closed eye (B). Image B Courtesy of Dr. Michael Blaivas.

for visualization of superficial structures. It is this type of probe that is best suited for bedside ophthalmic ultrasound in the emergency department. (Figure 2-2) Other uses include vascular access procedures and foreign body location.

• Specially designed **ophthalmic** probes are available. These probes are generally used with equipment designed to display both A-mode and B-mode results simultaneously. (Figure 2-3)

• **Curvilinear**, **annular**, and **phased array** transducers are also commonly found in the emergency department, but these generally operate on lower frequencies and are not well suited to ophthalmic ultrasound.

Beyond the Transducer

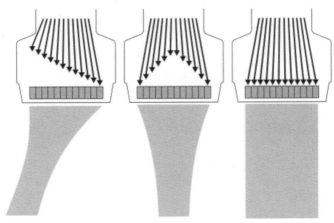

Figure 2-2 Electronic Linear Array Transducers. A large number of crystals are fired electronically to produce a sound beam from the probe. The focal length and direction of the beam can be changed by small differences in the sequence in which the crystals are fired.

In order for the transducer to function as part of the entire system, the ultrasound machine must generate, receive, interpret, and display information in the form of electrical impulses. The impulses generated from the transmitter are under control of the examiner in terms of the power and frequency of US waves desired from the transducer. When the echoed waves are received and transformed back into electrical impulses, they are fed to a receiver, which amplifies the information. The degree of amplification is also controlled by the examiner.

Finally, the converter takes the amplified data from the receiver and compiles it in order to form the images that are stored and displayed on the viewing monitor. The next section discusses more about how the scanner can both alter and interpret the image produced.

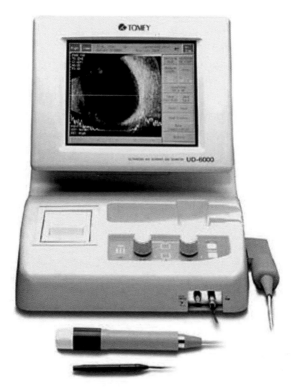

Figure 2-3 Transducers Utilized in the Ophthalmology Office. Ophthalmologists will generally use a specialized transducer that is only employed for evaluating the eye. The B-scan probe (top) has a marker dot for orientation. The A-scan probe (bottom) is smaller and provides an ice pick type image of the eye. Most ophthalmology probes, currently in use, perform A and B mode imaging. The B-scan ophthalmic probes usually can map A-mode information onto the B-mode image. The ophthalmological probes that are in direct contact with the eye and should be cleaned between patients with alcohol, bleach, Cidex or hydrogen peroxide and then rinsed with a wet cloth. If infection is suspected, it's best to cover the probe with small finger cots.

SECTION 3: EFFECTS AND ARTIFACTS

This section discusses controllable features of the US machine that allow for manipulation of the image. It is important to understand these fundamental concepts in order to obtain the best images. Also discussed are artifacts seen on images that are a result of the physics of the technology, not of structures being imaged.

Understanding the Formed Image

• **Gain** refers to the amplification applied to the signal received from the transducer. This has no effect on the sound waves transmitted by the ultrasound machine or those received by the transducer from the area of interest. Because the actual received amplitudes are very small, a certain degree of amplification is required in order to display an interpretable image. The amount of gain is easily controlled by the examiner. **Too little gain** will cause images to appear less echoic or darker than they actually are, and may render the images difficult to interpret. **Too much gain** will increase the apparent echogenicity or brightness of the structure being visualized, and perhaps create the illusion of a structure that does not exist. For example, an inappropriately high gain setting may create the appearance of diffuse

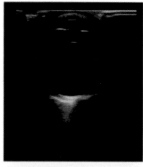

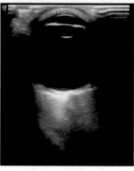

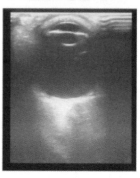

echogenic material within the normally anechoic vitreous, resembling a diffuse vitreous hemorrhage. To help set the appropriate gain setting, it may be helpful to also image the normal asymptomatic eye with the same gain settings and compare the image with the symptomatic eye. Ideally, the gain may be set objectively, according to the known sonodensity of a given structure, but in practice may be determined much more subjectively. In evaluating the posterior segment it is important to start with the higher gain settings to visualize any weak signals from vitreous opacities. Then the gain is

Figure 3-1 A-C Normal Eye with Different Gain Settings. A) Gain set too low. B) Proper gain settings. C) Excessive brightness. When scanning, the Sonographer will generally start with higher gain settings to identify less echogenic abnormalities, such as vitreous hemorrhage; then decrease the gain to more clearly identify more echogenic structures, such as retinal detachments.

decreased for better resolution of stronger echoes within the posterior segment from structures such as retina or choroid. (Figure 3-1 A-C)

• **Time Gain Compensation** - Because echoes farther from the probe provide a less intense signal than those close to the probe, a correction is needed to display similar echo strengths from given depths similarly. This is accomplished

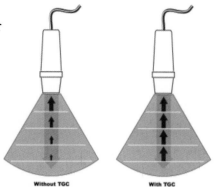

Figure 3-2 Time Gain Compensation (TGC). The TGC is normally set so that all parts of a homogeneous structure will have equivalent brightness. This is used to compensate for the loss of amplitude that occurs from the attenuation of sound waves as they pass through tissue. Most ultrasound machines allow the user to adjust the TGC to compensate for the degree of attenuation.

by time gain compensation. This feature allows a higher level of amplification to be applied to the farther fields within the image, allowing a structure with a constant sonodensity to be displayed with a constant echogenicity throughout the depth of the displayed image. Typically, one can adjust the relative gain throughout sections of the field by a series of sliders on the machine interface. (Figure 3-2)

• **Depth** is another controllable feature of the image displayed on the monitor. Ideally, the object of interest should be in the middle of the field being examined. For examination of the eye, the depth should be such that the globe takes up about two thirds of the displayed image.

Effects

The physical properties that define the interface between adjacent tissues or structures are responsible for the production of echoes that makes ultrasound imaging possible. However, the manner in which a sound wave strikes that interface may also produce effects or artifacts within the image, potentially confounding the interpretation

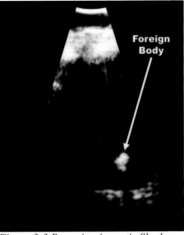

Figure 3-3 Posterior Acoustic Shadowing. This dense metallic foreign body in the orbit produces dark posterior shadowing deep to the foreign body.

of the images. While generally not as prevalent in ophthalmic ultrasound compared to abdominal imaging, the examiner should have an understanding of the principles that lead to these effects.

• **Posterior acoustic shadowing** occurs when the ultrasound beam contacts a highly reflective surface, prohibiting the majority of its energy from passing to deeper structures. This results in an echolucent stripe deep to the reflective structure. Dense metallic foreign bodies in the eye, calcium in a choroidal osteoma or retinoblastoma, optic nerve drusen and intraocular lens implants typically produce acoustic shadowing. (Figure 3-3)

Page 18

• **Lateral cystic shadowing**, also known as edge artifact, is cause by refraction of absorbed waves at the surface of a vessel or other cystic fluid-filled structure. This results in a relative absence of ultrasound waves in regions deep to the edge of the structure. This can be seen deep to both edges of the globe, but it is rarely otherwise mistaken for ocular pathology. (Figure 3-4)

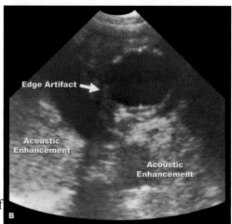

Figure 3-4 Acoustic Enhancement. This image depicts acoustic enhancement posterior to the fluid-filled structure between the two markers. There is also acoustic enhancement distal to the fluid that appears in the left portion of the image. Note that the wall of the structure between the markers demonstrates lateral cystic shadowing or edge artifact (arrow), which produces a thin dark shadow parallel to the direction of the ultrasound beam and tangential to the wall of the fluid-filled structure.

Artifacts

• The **mirror effect** may occur when the beam hits a reflective surface that is deep to a relatively echodense structure. Reflection of the beam may occur between the two, causes the image deep to the reflective surface to appear as a mirror image of that above it. This is best observed between the liver and diaphragm in abdominal scanning, but is of little significance to ophthalmic scanning.

• **Contact artifact** occurs when there is inadequate contact between the probe and the surface of the examined object or insufficient transmission medium (ultrasound gel).

• **Reverberation artifact** occurs when the beam passes through two highly reflective surfaces. The beam bounces back and forth between the two, resulting in horizontal bands of "reverberation echoes" that appear deep to the reflective surfaces. If the surfaces are very close together, the resulting reverberation echoes are stacked so that they appear as an echogenic stripe deep to the reflective surfaces, an artifact known as a "comet tail" pattern. (Figure 3-5 A&B)

• **Gain artifacts** are simply alterations in the image created by inappropriate gain settings, and are easily corrected with the appropriate gain or time gain compensation settings.

While these generally make interpretation of images more difficult, some effects and artifacts can be used to the advantage of the ultrasonographer. For example, metallic foreign bodies produce posterior acoustic shadowing or a reverberation artifact (i.e., bbs) that allows for ready identification within the otherwise echolucent vitreous humor. When an image does not appear as the examiner would have expected, effects and artifacts as described above should be considered as possible causes for

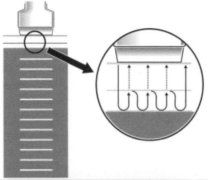

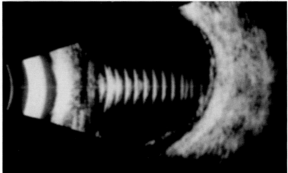

Figures 3-5 A&B Reverberation Artifact. A) This occurs when the ultrasound beam bounces back and forth between two reflective layers. Causes include inadequate gel, small hollow metallic foreign bodies and gas bubbles, amongst others. B) This patient had undergone a vitrectomy with fluid-gas exchange. Most of the gas had dissipated; however there were small bubbles present anteriorly producing this reverberation artifact. Note the retinal detachment present in this patient. Reprinted with permission from DiBernardo C, Schachat A, Fekrat S. Ophthalmic Ultrasound: A Diagnostic Atlas, New York, Thieme, 1998.

the distortion of the image.

SECTION 4: THE SONOGRAPHER

This section discusses the preparation and training recommended to obtain the most reliable information with bedside ophthalmic ultrasound.

Basic Training

It is recommended that before an emergency physician undergoes specific training in ophthalmic scanning, he or she have had a detailed training course in the use of emergency ultrasound as it applies to abdominal, pelvic and cardiac imaging. In contrast, the training of an ophthalmologist will be much more intensely focused on eye application and physics. A significant number of exams should be performed to the extent that the operator is comfortable using the equipment. Today, most emergency medicine and ophthalmology residency training programs are incorporating ultrasound training into their curriculum, and it is reasonable that graduates of such a program (or active trainees) may use the techniques described in this text successfully.

Ophthalmic Scanning Training

The goal of this text is to present ultrasound imaging as a useful adjunct to the emergency practitioner and ophthalmologist for the evaluation of potentially serious eye pathologies. Combining text review with hands-on training should be adequate to make this text useful for the practitioners.

Blaivas, et al. demonstrated that a group of residents and attending physicians were able to develop accurate ocular sonography skills after a brief formal training period. Sixty-one patients with a history of acute visual change or ocular trauma were assessed, and when compared with a standard of orbital CT and/or formal ophthalmologic consultation/exam, 60 of 61 interpretations were deemed accurate, of which 26 had significant intraocular pathology. This particular study was conducted in a large teaching hospital with a residency program and an active ultrasound training program. The resident training consisted of one hour of lecture and one hour of hands-on training dedicated to ocular ultrasonography. The attending physicians had no formal training but had performed between 15 and 75 ocular scans each. While this study is not without its limitations, it suggests that physicians and residents can perform these studies with good reliability after a relatively short training period.

By no means do we suggest that physicians with limited training can reliably exclude all potentially significant diagnoses, but we do believe bedside ultrasound can give the practitioner important information to correlate with other findings from the physical exam. For those who would desire further training than what can be done with books and bedside evaluations, it may be helpful to find an ophthalmologist with extensive ophthalmic ultrasound experience who may give further suggestions on examination techniques. (Figure 4-1 A&B)

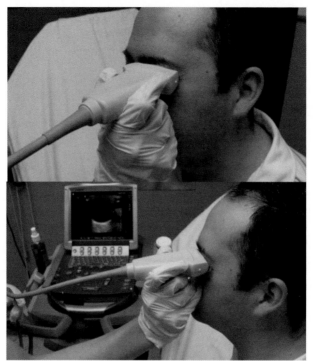

Figure 4-1 A&B Scanning with a Linear Array Transducer in the Emergency Department. A small to moderate amount of ultrasound gel is placed on top of the closed upper eyelid and a small parts probe is gently applied to the eyelid in the transverse plane. The ultrasound transducer is angled superiorly and gradually swept inferiorly in order to visualize the entire eye. Small changes in angulation result in large differences in the section being scanned. The patient is also asked to move their eye from left to right and from up to down in order to ensure that the entire orbit has been visualized. Sweeping the probe across the entire eye in the longitudinal plane can also be performed, if needed, to clarify the presence or absence of ocular pathology.

SECTION 5: SCANNING TECHNIQUES AND SAFETY CONSIDERATIONS

Equipment

While specialized ocular probes are available and used commonly in dedicated ophthalmologists' machines, they are rarely found in the emergency room. These are cylindrical probes, easily held in the hand like a pen, and have a small circular footprint meant to contact with the anesthetized eye surface. On dedicated ocular equipment, orientation to the monitor is different (near field to the left) and the marker dot toward the top of the image. Due to the relative infrequency of ED use, it is not often financially justified to purchase such probes for this setting. Today, however, many ED machines have a small parts probe. These are typically capable of frequencies from 5–15 MHz. This is the type of probe that would be most commonly used for ocular scanning, and is the best suited for ED use.

Scanning technique

- One primary advantage of ocular ultrasound in the ED setting is that it is **performed with a closed lid**. Often, patients with traumatic eye injuries are resistant to exam, lid manipulation, and may be photophobic. The closed-lid technique allows for rapid assessment without posing these problems to the patient.
- The patient may be examined in an **upright, semi-**

erect or supine position, depending on what the situation allows.

• The eye should be closed, and a generous amount of gel should be applied to the upper eyelid to ensure that proper contact and wave transmission are achieved.

• **Aftermovement**, indicative of mobility of a lesion, is determined by observing motion following cessation of rapid eye movement with B-mode scanning. Membranous structures such as vitreous or retinal detachments will display some aftermovement. More solid lesions such as choroidal detachments or tumors, do not display aftermovement. The movement observed with vitreous detachments is more prominent and "jiggly" than that seen with retinal detachments. This is nicely displayed with video at the following websites.

http://bjo.bmj.com/content/
suppl/2006/03/16/90.4.DC1/garciafinalfast.mov

http://www.ultrasoundvillage.com/imagelibrary/case
s/?id=6&media=108&testyourself=0

• **If there is suspicion but not an obvious ruptured globe, it is imperative that an adequate gel layer be used to avoid direct pressure on the eye**.

There are three basic orientations in which the globe can be scanned – transverse, longitudinal, and axial. (Figure 5-1 A&B)

• **Transverse** scanning is accomplished by orienting
the probe in a transverse plane with the eye everted
away from the probe.

• **Longitudinal** scans are done with the plane
perpendicular to the transverse plane, also with the
patient's gaze averted away from the probe. Gain-
ing the proper positioning for these types of scans is
more easily done with an ocular probe. Longitudinal scanning should also be attempted with a larger
footprint linear array transducer, when clarification
is needed.

• Finally the globe may be scanned with the probe
overlying the cornea with the gaze directed at the
probe. This is termed **axial** scanning. Adjustment of
the angle of the probe can result in less than perpendicular planes or **para-axial** scans. This is the easi-
est as it does not require as much cooperation on the
part of the patient to direct their gaze, which may be
painful or difficult in a given situation. (Figure 5-2)

• While in the hands of a skilled sonographer, transverse and longitudinal scanning methods are used to
eliminate the attenuation of sound beam penetration
by the lens. Limited examination time and larger
probe surface area may make axial and para-axial
scans more appropriate in emergency department.
Transverse axial and para-axial scanning is easier
to perform than longitudinal axial and para-axial
scanning with "large footprint" linear array probes.
Either way, scanning across (fanning motion) the

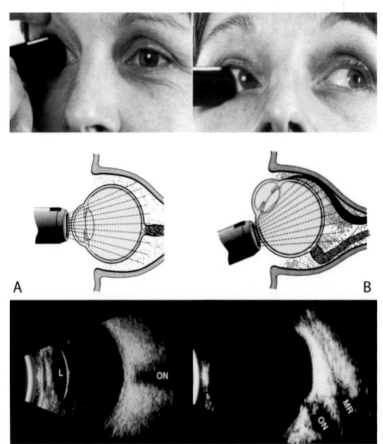

Figure 5-1 A&B Scanning using Ophthalmologic Equipment. A) B-mode scanning with probe in an axial plane creating two-dimensional acoustic section of the eye. B) B-mode scanning with the probe in a longitudinal plane bypassing the lens. The optic nerve in the image is represented by "ON" and medial rectus muscle by "MR". Reprinted with permission from Atta, H. Ophthalmic Ultrasound: A Practical Guide, New York, Churchill Livingstone, 1996.

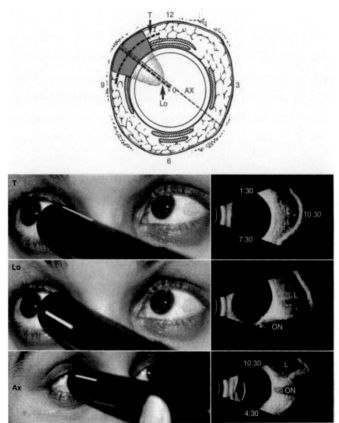

Figure 5-2 Imaging in Multiple Planes. The lesion can be visualized in multiple planes. Summing these images together allows one to map out the boarders of the lesion. The optic nerve in the images is represented by "ON" and the lesion by "L". Reprinted with permission from Byrne S, Green R. Ultrasound of the Eye and Orbit, 2nd ed. Philadelphia, PA: Mosby; 2002.

entire eye in perpendicular planes accompanied by movement of the eye to the upper and lower, left and right quadrants allows for a more thorough evaluation of the entire orbit.

Safety

Ultrasonography has long been safely used, even in relatively high frequencies, for a multitude of applications. While theoretical concerns exists about the effect that these high frequency waves may have on examined tissues, there is no evidence to support that there is any significant danger to the patient.

SECTION 6: EYE ANATOMY

This section will review the basic anatomy of the eye and briefly correlate the anatomy with its ultrasound findings. (Figures 6-1, 6-2)

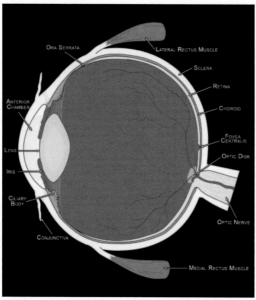

Figure 6-1 Normal eye. Anatomical Cross-Section of the Eye.

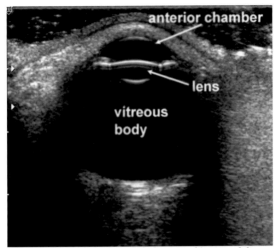

Fig 6-2 Normal Eye. Labeled ultrasound image of the normal eye. Image courtesy of Dr. Michael Blaivas.

Anterior elements

• The **cornea** is a layer of specialized epithelium that covers much of the visible anterior surface of the eye. This is responsible for the vast majority of the refraction necessary for visual acuity.

• The cornea is bordered by the **sclera**, covered anteriorly by the **bulbar conjunctiva**. This thick connective tissue layer surrounds the remainder of the eye. The border between the sclera and cornea is termed the **limbus**.

• Immediately posterior to the cornea is the **anterior chamber**, filled with aqueous humor. This is

normally an anechoic space on ultrasound.
- The anterior chamber is bordered posteriorly by the **iris**, which controls dilation of the **pupil**.
- Behind the iris lie the **ciliary body** peripherally, and the **lens** centrally. The contour and position of the lens can be readily identified with ED ultrasound.

Detailed visualization of the anterior chamber is possible with high frequency ocular probes (20-60 MHz), and is helpful in specialized settings in detecting pathology within the cilary body, cornea, iris, and within the anterior chamber itself. ED bedside scanning with a 7.5-15 MHz probe provides a limited

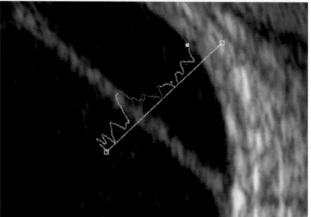

Figures 6-3 Echogenicity of the Retina, Choroid and Sclera. This patient with a retinal detachment clearly demonstrates the different echogenicity of the posterior structures; note that the retina and choroid is slightly less echogenic than the sclera. On A-mode scanning the height of the spike of the sclera > choroid > retina.

amount of detail of the anterior chamber, but may still be helpful in a limited number of scenarios (see Section 10). One should be able to visualize the corneal surface, the contour and depth of the anterior chamber, and the position of the lens.

Posterior elements

- Behind the anterior elements is the large, normally anechoic **vitreous chamber**. There are surrounding membranes that typically enclose this space that is generally only seen when pathologically separated from posterior layers. Collagen fibers extend throughout the vitreous and are attached around the optic nerve and are inserted in the peripheral retina near the ciliary body. These collagen fibers can sometimes be visualized when high enough gain is utilized.
- The first posterior layer of the eye (from anterior to posterior) is the **retina**, which is comprised of the specialized neuroepithelial photoreceptors. It is contiguous with the **optic nerve**.
- The **choroid** lies behind the retina and provides its vascular supply. It extends from the ciliary body anteriorly to the optic nerve posteriorly.
- The **sclera** lies behind the choroid and extends anteriorly to the cornea.

The majority of pathology that will be identified with ophthalmic ultrasound is in the posterior chamber. One should see a symmetric, spherical vitreous chamber that is anechoic. Posteriorly, the surface of the vitreous, the retina, choroid, and sclera

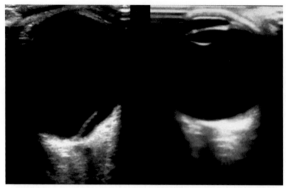

Figure 6-4 A&B Optic Nerve. A) Note the insertion of the retina into the optic nerve sheath in this patient with a retinal detachment. B) This normal optic nerve appears hypoechoic in comparison to the remainder of the posterior ocular tissues.

are in contact with each other. These structures may be difficult to distinguish from each other on B-mode scanning unless there is pathologic space between them. However, the retina/choroid is slightly less echogenic than the denser sclera and thus can occasionally be distinguished as a separate layer. The posterior eye should be a smooth surface without breaks, folds, or elevations. (Figure 6-3)

Extraocular elements

• The **extraocular muscles** are recognized as thin, straight, hypoechoic structures with insertion points on the globe. Evaluation of the extraocular muscles in cases of orbital cellulitis is discussed in Section 10.

• The **optic nerve** is hypoechoic in comparison to

the remainder of the extraocular tissues. (Figure 6-4 A&B) Identification of the optic nerve insertion into the globe will help to evaluate for other pathology. (Figure 6-4 A&B) Evaluation of the nerve sheath diameter is discussed in Section 10.

• The **central retinal** vessels can be evaluated with color Doppler imaging if the examiner has it available on his or her machine and is familiar with its use.

SECTION 7: THE POSTERIOR CHAMBER

Vitreous Hemorrhage

Vitreous hemorrhage can occur secondary to diabetic retinopathy, age-related macular degeneration, trauma, retinal vein occlusion, or retinal tears. The appearance of the vitreous hemorrhage (Figures 7-1 to 7-6) may differ depending both on the quantity of the hemorrhage and time course of the presentation.

Clinical Presentation

• Sudden onset of monocular visual acuity change, varying from multiple floaters to dark streaks in the visual field to light perception only. Degree of vision loss reflects both the amount and location of blood within the vitreous. Unless induced by trauma, this visual disturbance is usually painless.

• Traction of the vitreous against the adjacent retinal vessels leads to vascular leak or tear, with blood escaping into the vitreous gel. This may be related to a number of conditions, including diabetes (leading cause overall), central retinal vein occlusion, trauma (leading cause in younger patients) - including shaken baby syndrome, or subarachnoid hemorrhage (aka Terson's Syndrome, Figure 7-7, occurs in ~6% of SAH, usually younger patients).

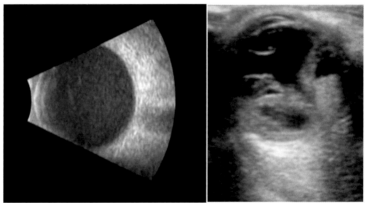

Figure 7-1 A&B Vitreous Hemorrhage. A) There is diffuse increased echogenicity of the vitreous secondary to the hemorrhage. This can be seen with venous occlusions, trauma, coagulopathy or secondary to neovascularization in diabetic retinopathy. B) This patient with a severe coagulopathy (INR > 8) developed vitreous hemorrhage without significant trauma. This patient presented with marked decrease in vision in the involved eye, a cloudy pupil and unilateral increased intraocular pressure. The vitreous hemorrhage was not initially apparent clinically, but was obvious on ultrasound examination. Note that there is layering of the hemorrhage present in this image. It appears that the bleeding caused the increased intraocular pressure in this case.

- No red reflex on direct ophthalmoscopy, although the lens appears to be clear and intact.

Ultrasound Findings

- Normal vitreous is not echogenic (except in the elderly, as below). In the early stages of vitreal hemorrhage, as blood leaks from the periphery, the vitreous will fill (or partially fill) with small dots and/or short lines of low reflectivity. If the gain is turned all the way up, vitreous fibers may become apparent as

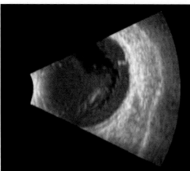

Figure 7-2 Vitreous Hemorrhage with Neovascularization in a Diabetic Patient. This patient demonstrates neovascularization which can mimic a shallow retinal detachment. This traction on the retinal vessels from diabetes leads to a vascular tear with leakage of blood into the vitreous gel. The small echogenic area on the retina may represent a prominent retina blood vessel from neovascularization or a small retinal detachment.

echogenic structures.

• The appearance of the hemorrhage may differ depending on the time course of the presentation. In general, more severe acute hemorrhage with clot formation is denser and has higher echogenicity. Chronic hemorrhage may become less echogenic

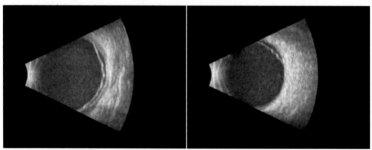

Figure 7-3 A&B Vitreous Hemorrhage with Shallow Retinal Detachments. This occurs commonly in the setting of diabetes (A&B) with neovascularization that scars and contracts over time putting traction on the retina. The vitreous hemorrhage is very apparent on direct ophthalmologic exam, however the posterior retinal detachment will not be visible with the ophthalmoscope and the ultrasound evaluation is very helpful in these cases.

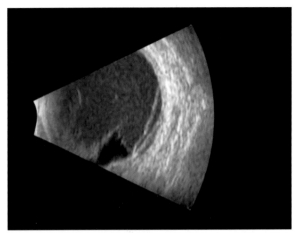

Figure 7-4 Vitreous Hemorrhage with Retinal and Choroidal Detachments. There is a moderate sized retinal detachment with a small deeper choroidal detachment and a large amount of vitreous hemorrhage. There is a small loculated area of normal vitreous fluid (black triangle).

and may display layering or organization. With time, the blood may clump into larger areas of distinct intra-vitreous opacities.

• The older blood from more severe hemorrhage may also settle to the dependent portion of the globe, forming a thicker, more sono-reflective (echogenic) layer or pseudomembrane in the vitreous. This may give an appearance similar to retinal detachment; however, the following characteristics distinguish pseudomembrane from vitreous hemorrhage. A pseudomembrane will taper as it extends superiorly. The edges of the pseudomembrane will disappear within the body of the vitreous, rather than having an

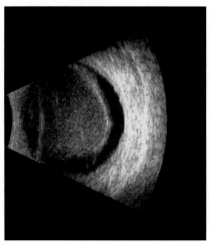

Figure 7-5 Vitreous Hemorrhage with Thickened Vitreous Membrane. The vitreous appears echogenic and the older detached vitreous membrane appears thicker. Over time the vitreous hemorrhage will become less echogenic.

insertion point into the fundus and the optic nerve.

• Elderly patients may display diffuse, evenly scattered echoes in their vitreous humor as a normal finding. However, these echoes are very lowly reflective and are usually not noticed unless the gain is increased above normal. In this instance, the examiner may confuse the echoes with the possibility of vitreous hemorrhage, but should remember to correlate findings to the clinical history and the opposite eye with similar gain settings.

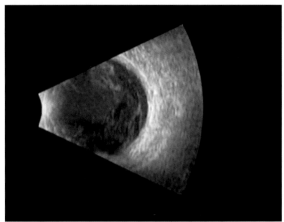

Figure 7-6 Vitreous Hemorrhage. The vitreous hemorrhage in this patient has varying degrees of echogenicity.

Management

• Early evaluation by an ophthalmologist is recommended for vitreous hemorrhage in cases of trauma (patient stability considered), severe coagulopathy, or when concomitant retinal tear/detachment is suspected.

• Urgent (within 24 hours) evaluation by an ophthalmologist is recommended in other cases. The ophthalmologist will evaluate the patient frequently to track the evolution or resolution of hemorrhage. It should be noted that vitreous hemorrhage may take over 3 months to completely resolve.

• Discharged patients should be instructed to sleep with the head elevated to 30-45°, so that the blood settles to the inferior pole of the globe. No clear benefit has been found to stopping aspirin therapy, although the decision to continue use of other anti-coagulants such as warfarin or clopidogrel should be left to the physician caring for the patient and the

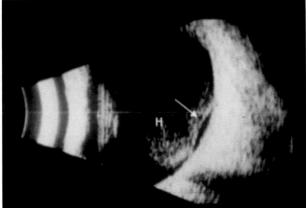

Figure 7-7 Terson's Syndrome - Intracranial Hemorrhage with Vitreous Hemorrhage. Following the intracranial hemorrhage, blood may tract into the vitreous along the central retinal vessels in the optic nerve sheath. Typically, there will be some hemorrhage layered over the posterior pole of the eye. There is a thin elevated membrane in the region of the macula which may represent a partial posterior vitreous detachment. Evaluation with an ophthalmoscope is limited because the vitreous hemorrhage obscures the retina. Reprinted with permission from DiBernardo C, Schachat A, Fekrat S. Ophthalmic Ultrasound: A Diagnostic Atlas, New York, Thieme, 1998.

ophthalmologist.

Structural Detachments

With the vitreous centrally, the periphery of the posterior globe is layered by the retina, the choroid, and the sclera (outermost), with the potential for separation or detachment between any two adjacent layers. Detachment is named for the inner layer of separation (e.g. - retinal detachment is retinal separation from the choroid, not the vitreous).

Understanding how the layers attach to each other is crucial to understanding how they will separate, and therefore, how they will appear with ultrasound imaging. Correlation to the clinical presentation is also essential to interpreting the images found on ultrasound.

Posterior Vitreous Detachment

Posterior Vitreous Detachment (PVD) can occur as a result of normal aging (benign condition of the aging eye), trauma, vitreous hemorrhage, or inflammation. In general, anything that increases vitreous opacity can contribute to contracture of the posterior membrane, causing it to detach from the retina. PVD (Figures 7-8 to7-12) may be very focal, may be extensive or complete. With partial detachments, points of attachment to the retina may be at sites of vitreoretinal adhesions. These usually occur at points of retinal neovascularization from retinal vein occlusion or diabetic retinopathy. The examiner may note a small degree of tractional retinal detachment at these sites.

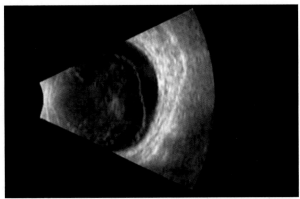

Figure 7-8 Posterior Vitreous Detachment. The thin, smooth, mobile membrane represents a posterior vitreous detachment. Rapid movement of the eye (after-movement) from one side to the other, results in significant wavelike, "jiggly" motion of the vitreous membrane. Low reflective vitreous opacities (vitreous syneresis) are frequently seen in the normal aging eye when the ultrasound gain is increased.

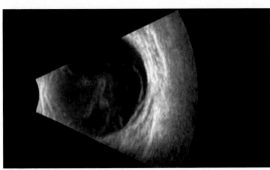

Figure 7-9 Posterior Vitreous Detachment with Retinal Detachment. Processes that increase vitreous opacity contribute to contracture of the posterior vitreous membrane resulting in its detachment from the retina. Occasionally there is tractional retinal detachment at sites of vitreoretinal adhesions as seen in this image.

Clinical Presentation

- Patient perceives monocular flashes or floaters as the contracting vitreous humor pulls on and then detaches from the retina.
- Small PVDs of gradual onset occur in every per-

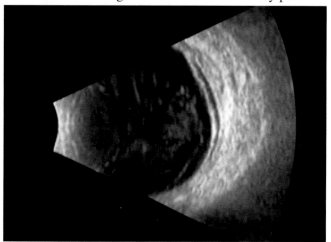

Figure 7-10 Posterior Vitreous Detachment with Retinal Detachment. The retinal detachment may have been precipitated by the vitreous detachment in this case. Echogenic vitreous densities from vitreous hemorrhage or inflammatory debris may be seen following vitreous and/or retinal detachments.

son eventually, with a mean onset at age 55.
- Larger PVDs of sudden onset occur concomitantly with vitreous hemorrhage, inflammatory processes, or other ocular abnormalities. These larger PVDs are more likely to present to the emergency department.

Ultrasound Findings

• As the edge of the vitreous separates from the retina, it is seen by ultrasound as a thin, smooth, and somewhat mobile membrane. Movement of the eye should result in a wave-like motion of the membrane. The membrane may be slightly thicker in the presence of hemorrhage or inflammatory debris lying adjacent to the detached membrane.

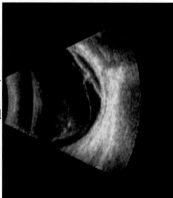

Figure 7-11 Retinal Detachment with Posterior Vitreous Detachment. The vitreous detachment inserts directly on the retinal causing the retinal detachment.

• The vitreous usually holds firm to the retina at the ora serrata. There may be attachment at the optic nerve head, but it is much less strongly adherent than the retina, and may often not be attached. With complete detachment from the optic nerve head, one may note a Weiss ring, which is a small ring of tissue (two small densities in cross section) that usually anchors the membrane to the optic nerve head.

• Chronic PVD may become more stiff and dense and may resemble retinal detachment. Differentiation may be difficult and may depend on specialized examination and A-mode correlation.

• Vitreous detachments tend to demonstrate very "jiggly" motion with aftermovement that is more prominent than what is seen with retinal detach-

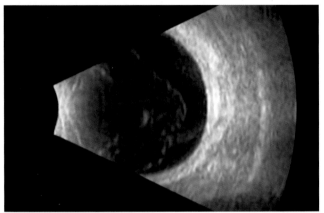

Figure 7-12 Posterior Vitreous Detachment. The patients often perceive flashes or floaters as the contracting vitreous separates from the retina in the involved eye. The vitreous is thinner, more mobile and less echogenic than the retina.

ments.

Management

- Usually a benign finding, with symptom resolution as floaters descend below the axis of sight.
- Patients should be referred to an ophthalmologist for follow-up of the conditions that may predispose them to more significant visual disturbances such as an underlying small retinal tear.

Retinal Detachment

There are a number of potential etiologies for retinal detachments. These include subretinal fluid accumulation (blood from trauma or tumor, or exudate from uveal effusion or inflamma-

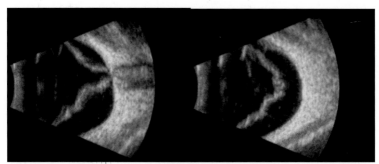

Figure 7-13 A&B Retinal Detachment. A) This image demonstrates a classical funnel shaped retinal detachment that remains attached at the optic nerve sheath. Note the anechoic appearance of the optic nerve sheath. If the macula is detached, the chance for recovery of vision is small. The retinal attachment at the optic nerve sheath is very strong and is disrupted very rarely in the setting of severe trauma. B) Image from the same patient with a retinal detachment where the plane of imaging does not include the optic nerve sheath.

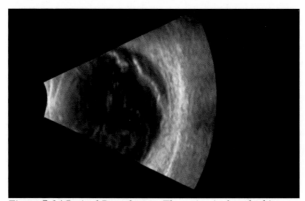

Figure 7-14 Retinal Detachment. The retina is detached in the superior temporal field. This image also demonstrates a separation or tear in the retina.

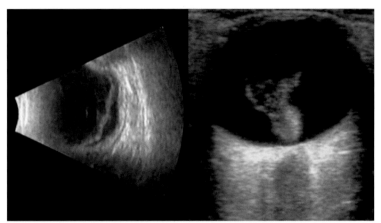

Figure 7-15 A&B Chronic Retinal Detachment. A) This image demonstrates a chronic retinal detachment with thickening of the retina, choroid and sclera. When assessing for aftermovement, retinal detachments are much less mobile than vitreous detachments. B) This chronic retinal detachment demonstrates significant retinal thickening. Chronic retinal detachments are less mobile with eye movement than acute retinal detachments.

tion), traction (from diabetic disease or trauma), or tears. Usually, the sonographic appearance is characteristic. (Figures 7-13 to 7-18)

Clinical Presentation

- Initial symptoms may involve the perception of flashing lights or showering visual floaters. The classically described "falling curtain" or "black veil" visual deficit develops over several hours to a few days. Visual acuity will be markedly disturbed if the area of detachment includes the macula.
- 3 mechanisms are described by which the retina

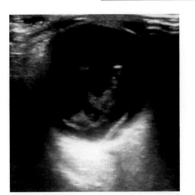

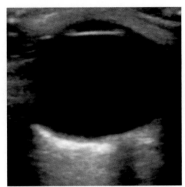

Figure 7-16 Retinal Detachment with Vitreous Hemorrhage. One can see the retinal detachment's insertion at the optic nerve sheath. In addition, there is vitreous hemorrhage present.

Figure 7-17A Retinal Detachment. The detachment is not visualized on the initial imaging with the patient looking straight ahead.

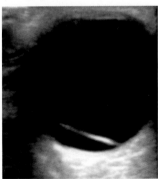

Figure 7-17B Retinal Detachment. The patient from 7-17A looks to one side and then looks up and down the detachment becomes obvious. This retinal detachment occurred in a near-sighted patient. Near-sightedness predisposes to rhegmatogenous retinal detachments.

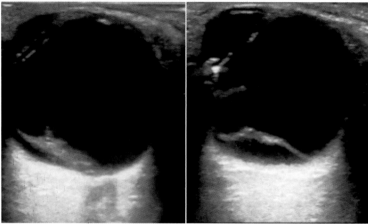

Figure 7-18 A&B Thicker Appearance of Retinal Detachment. A) This retinal detachment appears thicker as a result of viewing it obliquely down the length of the detachment. B) When viewed at a slightly different angle, the retinal detachment appears thinner, more in line with the typical retinal detachment. Rhegmatogenous retinal detachments (tears) represent an ocular emergency and occur more commonly in middle-aged or older patients with severe myopia (near-sightedness).

separates from the choroid:

    o **Rhegmatogenous (tearing) detachment** occurs when a spontaneous tear in the retina allows vitreous fluid to enter, separating the tissue layers. This is the most common mechanism of retinal detachment.

    o **Tractional detachment** occurs when the vitreous humor contracts, but remains tightly adherent to the retina. This may be a complication of diabetic retinopathy, sickle cell disease, or simply increasing age.

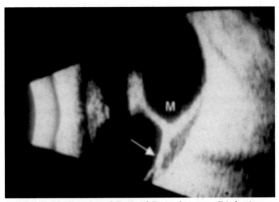

Figure 7-19 Tractional Retinal Detachments. Diabetic patients frequently have vitreous hemorrhage and multiple membranes that can result in tractional detachment. The arrow points to region of tent-like traction on the retina. Reprinted with permission from DiBernardo C, Schachat A, Fekrat S. Ophthalmic Ultrasound: A Diagnostic Atlas, New York, Thieme, 1998.

o **Exudative detachment** occurs when subretinal fluid accumulates without any break in the retina. This is usually related to either a severe inflammatory/infectious process or the development of a tumor within the eye and is relatively rare.

• Risk factors include myopia (nearsightedness), previous ocular surgery (especially cataract surgeries), and trauma (including a variety of sports and activities such as boxing and bungee jumping). Surgery or trauma may be several months prior to the development of the retinal detachment. Other medical conditions associated with retinal detachment include diabetes, a variety of non-ocular cancers, sickle cell disease, eclampsia, and prematurity. (Figure 7-19)

• Only the most dramatic cases of detachment may be observed with direct ophthalmoscopy – the clearly elevated, gray-hued retina will appear in marked contrast to the rest of the retinal tissue. Most cases, however, will be difficult to diagnosis by direct ophthalmoscopy or other techniques practiced by emergency physicians.

Ultrasound Findings

• When the retina separates from the choroid, it is recognized as a brightly echogenic membrane, tethered at the optic disc and ora serrata, where the retina is most firmly attached. The motion is more restricted than that of PVD, as the retina is more strictly tethered. Mobility decreases more with increasing time from detachment. Thus acute changes in vision as a result of retinal detachment should have a somewhat mobile membrane visualized.

o   Always take note of the points of apparent insertion. These should not change as the patient moves the eye or as the examiner scans from multiple angles.

o   The retina may rarely undergo complete detachment in cases of severe trauma.

• When detached, the retina may be perceived as a taut, smooth membrane, but more often has a folded

appearance within the vitreous, somewhat similar
to a PVD. However, when scanned from multiple
angles, and with the patient moving the eye, the retinal structure demonstrates minor changes in form,
unlike the more fluid, "jiggly" appearing PVD.

> o   In the case of detachment secondary to a
> large retinal tear, the membrane can appear
> somewhat more fluid.

• Extensive detachments may appear funnel- or
T-shaped. The three dimensional form of the retina
will not change much as the patient moves the eye.
In this setting the retina generally remains attached
at the optic nerve.

• Tractional detachments occur as a result of a
vitreoretinal adhesion, usually as a result of diabetes.
Small adhesions will lift the retina at a single point
and result in a tent-like appearance, while larger adhesions lift a larger portion of the retina and result in
a table-top appearance. Tractional detachments may
vary greatly in magnitude, from subtle elevations in
the retina to frank focal detachments.

Management

• Rhegmatogenous retinal detachment is one of the
most time critical eye emergencies encountered in
the emergency department. With rapid diagnosis
and treatment, a patient can truly have their vision
saved from what was once a uniformly blinding
condition.

• Rhegmatogenous retinal detachment requires

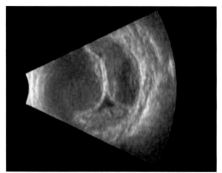

Figure 7-20 Choroidal Detachment. There are multiple hemorrhagic "kissing" choroidal detachments present in this image. These most commonly occur intra- or postoperatively. With aftermovement (rapid movement of the eyes from side to side) one may visualize spinning of the echogenic blood components inside the choroidal detachment. There is only a small amount of dark triangle shaped normal vitreous in this image.

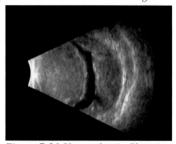

Figure 7-21 Hemorrhagic Choroidal Detachment. Multiple hemorrhagic choroidal detachments are visualized in this patient.

Page 58

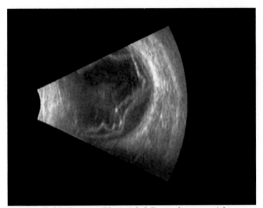

Figure 7-22 Serous Choroidal Detachment with
a Retinal Detachment. This patient has a serous
(anechoic fluid below) choroidal detachment that
probably caused the secondary retinal detachment.
The choroidal detachment may have been hemor-
rhagic initially and became progressively more serous
over time.

prompt ophthalmologic intervention if the macula is
still attached. If the macula is detached as seen with
more extensive retinal detachments, surgery may be
delayed for 72 hours or more. Operative intervention may be futile in patients where the visual acuity
is decreased to the point of motion perception only
as a result of the detachment (non-salvageable);
however, coexistent vitreous hemorrhage with retinal
detachment can result in marked decreased visual
acuity that may be correctable.

Choroidal Detachment

Choroidal detachments can be the result of several conditions, including idiopathic, inflammatory, post-surgical (most common), and traumatic. They occur when serous fluid, blood or inflammatory debris accumulates in the suprachoroidal space. (Figures 20-22)

Clinical Presentation

• As the choroid is firmly attached to the sclera, only a few conditions will allow for their separation. A serous exudate filling the potential space between these layers may occur with inflammatory conditions, or when systemic blood pressure greatly exceeds intraocular pressure. Similarly, transmural pressure may increase during a Valsalva maneuver, leading to choroidal detachment. Hemorrhage may also lead to the separation of the choroid and the sclera, although this is most commonly a post-surgical event, and rarely directly related to trauma. Choroidal detachment is only rarely a spontaneous event.

• Serous choroidal detachments are usually painless, with varying degrees of visual loss. Hemorrhagic choroidal detachments are described as throbbing and painful with an immediate severe vision loss. In both cases, the choroid usually separates at the periphery, and the degree of visual disturbance reflects the detached membrane interrupting the visual axis.

Ultrasound Findings

• They are usually peripheral, and have a character-istic smooth, dome shaped appearance, with possible echogenicity in the suprachoroidal space, depending on the cause (blood or inflammatory debris will be echogenic).

• There is usually no significant choroidal mobility seen on kinetic exam.

• As the detachment spreads circumferentially, the detached membrane appears as two detachments in apposition. Larger detachments may even show the membranes centrally meeting, giving an hourglass shaped appearance on scanning. They may have a bullous or scalloped appearance, and will insert posteriorly near, but not into, the optic disc. This is in contrast to retinal detachments, which will insert directly into the disc.

• Additional challenge is presented when faced with a less elevated choroidal detachment which can ap-pear more like a retinal detachment with respect to its shape and mobility. Alternatively, chronic retinal detachments become thicker and less mobile over time. A history of the patient's prior visual problems and the location of insertion help differentiate these conditions.

Management

• Choroidal detachment has a significant prognosis for lasting visual deficit. All cases should be dis-cussed with an ophthalmologist to determine appro-

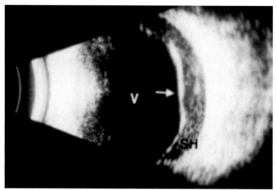

Figure 7-23 Subvitreal Hemorrhage. This image demonstrates totally clear (anechoic) vitreous with a dense posterior vitreous detachment (arrow) with subvitreal (subhyaloid hemorrhage - SH) hemorrhage. Reprinted with permission from DiBernardo C, Schachat A, Fekrat S. Ophthalmic Ultrasound: A Diagnostic Atlas, New York, Thieme, 1998.

priate care. Intraocular pressure should be reported to the ophthalmologist, in order to determine the appropriate combination of medications to be taken until the patient can be seen.

• Ultimate care may include surgical drainage of the hemorrhage or serous collection.

Other Findings of Non-Acute Disease

While evaluating the eye for acute pathology, the sonographer may encounter other findings that may or may not be related to the patient's trauma or acute visual change. These findings are mentioned only so that their appearance is not mistaken for other pathology.

Non-Hemorrhagic Vitreous Opacities

Not all vitreous opacities represent hemorrhage. Other etiologies include inflammatory or infectious material as seen in uveitis or endophthalmitis. Often these can be differentiated from blood on a clinical basis. Asteroid hyalosis is a chronic condition resulting in a deposition of calcium soaps within the vitreous. This has a characteristic appearance of bright, point-like echogenicities with an area of clear vitreous separating these densities from the posterior hyaloid. Vitreous cysts, appearing as ring-like echogenicities, may be congenital or pathologic. A

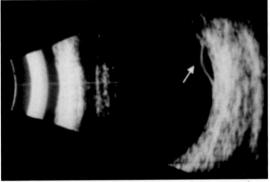

Figure 7-24 Retinoschisis. This patient demonstrated bilateral, shallow, elevated membranes in the far temporal regions. Many patients with this condition are asymptomatic, but they may become symptomatic in very advanced cases. The relative thinness of the membrane, location and the small dome-shape supports retinoschisis versus other types of detachments. Reprinted with permission from DiBernardo C, Schachat A, Fekrat S. Ophthalmic Ultrasound: A Diagnostic Atlas, New York, Thieme, 1998.

dense nodule within the cyst may suggest intraocular cysticerco-sis.

Submembranous Hemorrhage

Subvitreal hemorrhage or subretinal hemorrhage may occur with PVD or RD, respectively. Blood in the subvitreal space behaves differently than vitreous hemorrhage in that it does not easily clot and will often remain mobile within the space (posterior hyphema). Examination in the erect and supine position may illustrate this finding. (Figure 7-23)

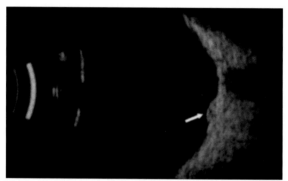

Figure 7-25 Macular Degeneration – Disciform Macular Lesion (wet degeneration). There is a moderately elevated, dome-shaped, heterogeneous, echogenic lesion in the region of the macula (arrow). There are two forms of age-related macular degeneration: wet and dry. Dry degeneration results in atrophy which is often not visible on ultrasound. In long standing cases of dry degeneration, there may be areas of calcification in the minimally elevated retina that might occasionally be seen with ultrasonography. The wet form results in disciform lesions as demonstrated in this image and is usually associated with more significant vision loss. Reprinted with permission from Byrne S, Green R. Ultrasound of the Eye and Orbit, 2nd ed. Philadelphia, PA: Mosby; 2002.

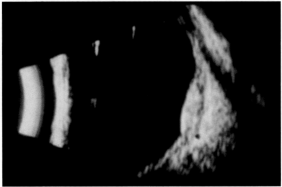

Figure 7-26 Hemangioma. Choroidal hemangiomas appear as solid, dome-shaped, homogeneous structures that are echogenic and usually located at the posterior pole. Reprinted with permission from DiBernardo C, Schachat A, Fekrat S. Ophthalmic Ultrasound: A Diagnostic Atlas, New York, Thieme, 1998.

Retinoschisis

Retinoschisis occurs when layers within the retina separate from each other. The disease may occur as an X-linked condition (presenting in school-aged boys) or as a non-genetic condition affecting the elderly. The condition is often bilateral, and it commonly occurs in the infero-temporal portions of the fundus. Hemorrhage may occur between the separating layers of the retina. While retinoschisis is not described as a cause of acute visual loss, it may be seen while examining the eye for other purposes, and it is important to distinguish from other conditions, especially retinal and/or choroidal detachments.

Retinoschisis is noted as a very thin, dome-shaped membrane protruding from the infero-temporal portion of the retina.

Page 65

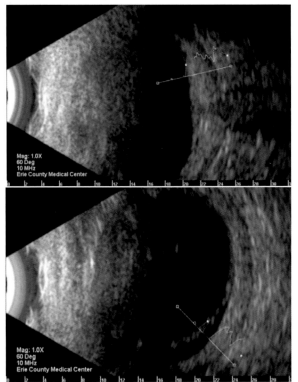

Figure 7-27 A&B Choroidal Thickening. A) Chronic hypotonia predisposes the patient to choroidal thickening. B) Choroidal thickening can also occur in the setting of a chronic retinal detachment.

Echogenic hemorrhage may be noted posteriorly. The differentiation of retinoschisis from other detaching layers is largely made based on the clinical history. However, in confounding cases, the examiner should look at the relative thinness of the membrane, the location, and the classic small dome shape that typifies

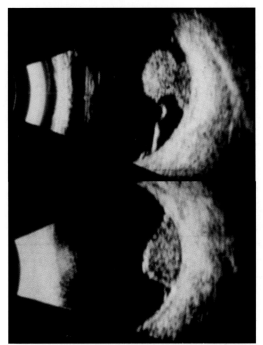

Figure 7-28 A&B Melanomas. A) When a melanoma breaks through Bruch's membrane a "collar button" appearance may occur as demonstrated in this case. These may vary in size and configuration depending on the location of rupture. B) On ultrasound, a melanoma appears as a solid (or collar button), vascular (shimmering within lesion), dome-shaped lesion of low to medium echogenicity. Reprinted with permission from DiBernardo C, Schachat A, Fekrat S. Ophthalmic Ultrasound: A Diagnostic Atlas, New York, Thieme, 1998.

retinoschisis compared with other detachments.

Retinoschisis is a chronic condition and most patients will already be following with an ophthalmologist. Most patients with retinoschisis are asymptomatic, but this condition may be associated with large peripheral field defects in advanced cases. If there is any concern or confusion over the exact etiology of a visualized membrane, an ophthalmologist should be consulted. (Figure 7-24)

Macular Degeneration

It is important to recognize the appearance of age-related wet macular degeneration as it may be noted while searching for other potential acute pathology. Subretinal exudate, hemorrhage, and subsequent fibrosis and calcification can result in a mildly elevated disciform, dome-shaped lesion. Imitators may include nevus, hemangioma, and metastatic lesions. All should be followed by an ophthalmologist. (Figures 7-25, 7-26)

Choroidal Thickening

Thickening of the choroid may be caused by low intra-ocular pressure, inflammation, chronic retinal detachment or infiltration. It may be associated with lymphoid hyperplasia, lymphoma, uveal effusion, sarcoid, Lyme disease, or phthisis. Correlation with A-scan is very beneficial in distinguishing the retinochoroid layer from the sclera, and in further quantifying the amount of thickening. This having been mentioned, in the absence of other focal pathology or detachment, choroidal thickening alone would likely be difficult for the EP to diagnose, and would likely not contribute to the diagnosis or care of acute visual change or traumatic injury. (Figure 7-27)

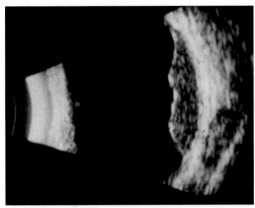

Figure 7-29 Metastatic Cancer. The ultrasound appearance of metastatic carcinoma to the choroid is a minimally elevated lesion with an irregular surface often with central excavation. Reprinted with permission from DiBernardo C, Schachat A, Fekrat S. Ophthalmic Ultrasound: A Diagnostic Atlas, New York, Thieme, 1998.

Tumors

While tumors should not be causes of acute visual disturbance, they may also be seen on examination. There are multiple appearances, and they can occur in many locations. While complete sonographic evaluation of these is not prudent in the emergency setting, referral should be made for any abnormal finding not explained by another diagnosis. (Figures 7-28 to 7-30)

SECTION 8: TRAUMA

While several of the previously discussed findings have both non-traumatic and traumatic etiologies, there are a number of pathologic findings that ultrasound can help the physician diagnose that have trauma as the sole cause. This section describes some of those findings.

Ruptured Globe

With either blunt or penetrating trauma, the sclera can become disrupted, resulting in an open or ruptured globe. Typically, severe injuries resulting in obvious globe ruptures need no further diagnostic care unless an intraocular foreign body is suspected. When the diagnosis is clearly apparent, ophthalmologic consultation should be sought immediately without delay for ultrasonography. CT may be necessary for foreign body identification, but can be done after notification is made. Ultrasound may be used to confirm the diagnosis of globe rupture. While ultrasound may not detect the actual rupture, several echographic clues can assist in the diagnosis, including hemorrhage in the immediate episcleral space, a thickened or detached choroid, a detached retina in the area of concern, vitreous hemorrhage and a scleral buckling. An advantage of ultrasound is that it can be performed without the discomfort associated with a thorough eye exam.(Figures 8-1 A&B, 8-2)

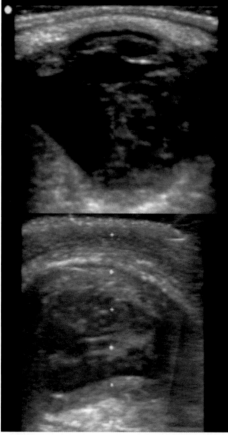

Figure 8-1 A&B Ruptured Globe. A) As a result of an injury from a BB gun and B) scissors. Note the loss of architecture, loss of anterior chamber, presence of vitreous hemorrhage and flattening of the globe in these patients. Images courtesy of Fernando Lopez M.D.

Clinical Presentation

- Physical exam findings include pain, severe visual deficit, limitation of extraocular motion, possible visualization of prolapsed pigmented uveal tissue or vitreous and decreased eye pressure.

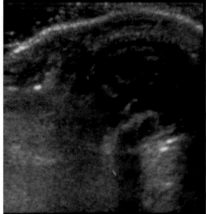

Figure 8-2 Ruptured Globe. There is gross distortion of the architecture, flattening of the globe and significant vitreous hemorrhage.

Ultrasound Findings

- Globe rupture leads to posterior scleral buckling, flattening of the anterior chamber or vitreous hemorrhage. In addition, extrusion of the vitreous fluid or retina through the rupture site may be visualized. Blunt trauma may lead to posterior scleral rupture in some cases.

- In penetrating injury, vitreous hemorrhage in the tract of the penetration will either lead to the foreign body retained within the globe, or will follow through to the exit wound through the posterior sclera.

- A scleral fold may result from penetrating or blunt trauma secondary to decompression and collapse of the scleral wall.

- **Examination *must* be done with adequate gel**

and only the minimal amount of pressure against the globe needed to acquire images. An appropriate gel layer generally allows for negligible pressure application. Any excessive force may lead to extrusion of intraocular contents from the globe.

• Periorbital or intraocular air may be another finding noted with significant trauma.

Management

• Emergent ophthalmologic consultation is indicated.

• CT scanning should be performed if necessary to rule out a foreign body, even if not seen on ultrasound examination.

• Tetanus prophylaxis and antibiotics are indicated.

Penetrating Foreign Body

Often the penetration of foreign bodies is apparent from the history and external examination of the eye. In other cases, the determination may be more difficult, and symptoms at the time of injury and at the time of presentation may differ and perhaps improve. (Figure 8-3)

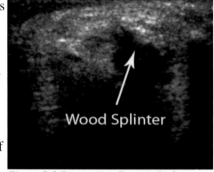

Wood Splinter

Figure 8-3 Penetrating Foreign Body. There is a piece of wood (arrow) embedded in the orbit of this patient. Note the dark posterior shadowing deep to the superficial foreign body in the center of the image. There is also echogenic hemorrhage/clot apparent on both sides of the foreign body.

Clinical Presentation

- Although symptoms may have lessened since the traumatic event, a patient with a suggestive patient history merits evaluation.

Ultrasound Findings

- Ultrasound detection of foreign bodies is highly variable according to the material of which the foreign body is composed, as well as its size and orientation.
- Small penetrating foreign bodies may create an isolated tract of hemorrhage within the vitreous.
- Metallic foreign bodies are highly echogenic and easily detected in most cases, often with posterior shadowing. Spherical metals, such as BB's, can pro-

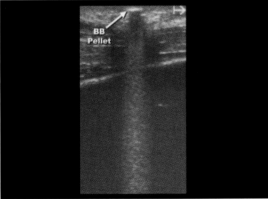

Figure 8-4 Metallic Foreign Body. This hollow BB pellet creates an echogenic line at the metal-soft tissue interface and comet tail shadowing deep to the BB pellet.

duce a great deal of comet-tail artifact. (Figure 8-4)

• Glass shards can be more difficult to detect. The sound waves must strike perpendicular to a flat surface on the glass in order to be reflected back to the probe. Scanning should be done from multiple angles to detect the true placement and size of the piece(s) of glass.

• Organic matter, such as wood, will have varying degrees of echogenicity, although they are generally highly reflective in the immediate post-traumatic period.

• As an object penetrates the eye, it may introduce eyelashes or small air bubbles into the tract of penetration. Eyelashes produce a bright signal without shadowing. Air bubbles may produce a signal suggestive of a solid foreign body, but the signal moves within the globe as the patients head is placed in various positions, owing to the lower density of the air. These air bubbles usually resolve in just a few days after the insult.

• Some materials do not have the echogenicity required for ultrasound evaluation. Also, foreign bodies may be difficult to detect when they sit adjacent to the retina. Always correlate ultrasound findings with the history, the examination by direct ophthalmoscopy, and other radiographic modalities.

• Although ultrasound can facilitate the diagnosis of intraocular foreign body, even the "easily detectable" metallic foreign body may be missed on ultrasound. One case report (Prakash, G. et al) is given of an instance when a metallic foreign body was immediately overlying the optic disc, thus making it impossible to distinguish shadowing from the posterior-lying optic nerve.

Management
• Any intra-ocular foreign body detected or very strongly suggested by history mandates consultation with an ophthalmologist. Tetanus vaccination and antibiotic administration may be indicated as well.

Lens Subluxation or Dislocation
The lens suspended behind the pupil by zonular fibers, and sufficiently larger than the pupil that even in a widely dilated eye, the outer rim of the lens cannot be seen. Blunt trauma to the eye can stretch or rupture the zonular fibers, resulting in partial (subluxation) or complete dislocation of the lens.

When the posterior lens capsule is disrupted from (usually blunt) trauma, the lens may either become subluxed or completely dislocated. If the patient is awake, one would expect a visual change related to the degree of subluxation or dislocation. Lens dislocation should be readily visualized on ultrasound exam as the lens will move toward the dependent portion of the vitreous chamber. (Figure 8-5 A&B, 8-6)

Clinical Presentation
• Visual acuity will be greatly affected by malposition of the lens. If the patient is able to open the eye and the pupil is dilated, the edge of the lens may be noted on direct ophthalmoscopy. However, in the

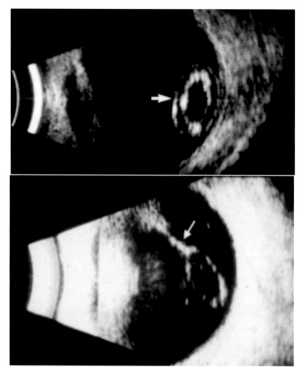

Figure 8-5 A&B Dislocated Lens. A) This image shows the oval shaped lens (arrow) on the surface of the retina following a blunt traumatic injury to the eye. In addition, there are significant cataractous changes to the lens. If the lens ruptures (not in this case), there may be extrusion of lens material into the vitreous and an irregular contour to the lens. Reprinted with permission from Byrne S, Green R. Ultrasound of the Eye and Orbit, 2nd ed. Philadelphia, PA: Mosby; 2002. B) The echolucent dislocated lens in the vitreous cavity is suspended by a hemorrhagic membrane (arrow). Reprinted with permission from DiBernardo C, Schachat A, Fekrat S. Ophthalmic Ultrasound: A Diagnostic Atlas, New York, Thieme, 1998.

setting of acute trauma, such an examination may not be feasible.
• Patients may complain of monocular decrease in visual acuity or a monocular diplopia.

Ultrasound Findings
• Owing to the more anterior nature of the lens, it is best imaged with higher frequency probes.
• The lens should be readily identifiable by its shape

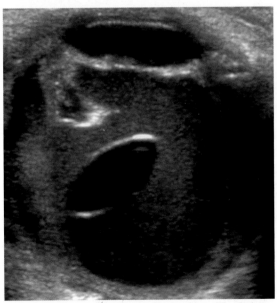

Figure 8-6 Dislocated Lens with Vitreous Hemorrhage. The dislocated lens is seen floating in the vitreous cavity in this patient with significant blunt trauma directly to the eye. The lens is prominently outlined by the large amount of vitreous hemorrhage. Courtesy of Dr. Donna D'Souza.

and size. The formation of cataracts may increase
the echogenicity of the lens itself. (Figures 8-7, 8-8)
• Subluxation or dislocation is noted simply as a
matter of the appearance of the lens anywhere other
than its normal position directly behind the pupil. It
may be subluxed anteriorly, laterally, or slightly posteriorly. If the lens has completely dislocated, it is
usually found floating deep in the vitreous substance

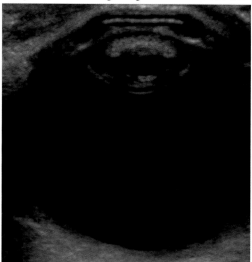

*Figure 8-7 Cataract. This advanced cataract appears echogenic on ultrasound
examination. A cataract forms as a result of progressive painless clouding of
the lens. This may occur from aging (most commonly), post traumatic, diabetes,
radiation and occasionally may be congenital. Visual deterioration occurs with
increasing severity of the cataract. Ocular ultrasound allows one to evaluate
the posterior aspect of the eye when the opaque lens obscures normal visualization of the retina with an ophthalmoscope. Courtesy of Dr. Donna D'Souza.*

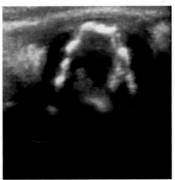

Figure 8-8 Severe Chronic Cataract. This patient has complete opacification of the lens and regions adjacent to the lens. These opacified areas appear strongly echogenic on ultrasound examination.

or sliding along the surface of the retina.

• A grossly misshapen lens after severe blunt trauma suggests lens capsule rupture.

Management

• Subluxation or complete dislocation of the lens mandates referral to an ophthalmologist. Concomitant injuries to the globe often necessitate immediate evaluation, as well.

Hyphema

A hyphema is a clinical diagnosis readily made by direct examination of the eye with blood within the normal clear anterior chamber.

Clinical Presentation

• Blunt trauma to the eye may result in blood seeping into the anterior segment of the eye. On direct examination, the blood is visualized anterior to the iris, settling in the gravity dependent portion of the anterior chamber.

• With significant swelling of the eyelids, it may be difficult to assess the presence of a hyphema. In this situation, ultrasound may be helpful. More importantly, a hyphema may prevent adequate direct ophthalmoscopic examination of the posterior segment, necessitating the use of ultrasound for complete eye evaluation.

Ultrasound Findings

• Because hyphema is a pathology related to the anterior segment, evaluation is best done with a step-off technique or a higher frequency probe, as previously described. This finding can be easily missed if using a lower frequency probe without a step-off technique.

• The normally clear anterior chamber will be (partially) filled with echogenic material, settling to the gravity dependent portions of the eye. (See Figure 10-3)

Management

• Glaucoma is the major potential complication secondary to a hyphema. When the erythrocytes are trapped in the canals of Schlemm, aqueous outflow is obstructed, leading to increased pressure in the anterior segment of the eye.

• The patient should be placed in a semi-erect position of approximately 45 degrees. The upright posture allows the erythrocytes to settle inferiorly, while aqueous continues to flow in the superior portions of the anterior chamber. The slightly reclined position helps to prevent the blood from staining the cornea.

• Emergent ophthalmologic consultation should be sought. Instructions for activity restrictions to help prevent rebleeding are crucial.

Peripheral Retinal Dialysis

In severe blunt trauma, retinal detachment may occur to a greater degree than typically seen. As mentioned, before, attachment of the retina to the ora serrata peripherally is strong. In peripheral retinal dialysis (PRD), the retina becomes detached from the ora serrata and is seen floating loosely, untethered, except at the optic nerve. Beyond this, the appearance is similar to other large retinal detachments.

SECTION 9: EXTRAOCULAR PATHOLOGY

Optic Nerve Sheath Measurement in Elevated ICP

One of the potentially promising applications of ultrasound scanning of the optic nerve is in respect to the relationship of the nerve/sheath diameter to intracranial pressure (ICP). While clinical measures in combination with CT scanning are the usual means of diagnosis (and direct measurement via ventriculostomy the gold standard), ultrasound may prove as a useful tool to direct therapy if CT scanning is unavailable or delayed. An example may be a mass casualty situation in which timely CT of patients is not feasible. Also, in rural facilities where emergent neurosurgical consultation is not available and CT scanning would only delay transport to the appropriate facility, rapid bedside ultrasound (which may already be at the bedside for a FAST exam in trauma patients) may be a means to direct ICP-lowering therapy without delaying transport. There exists a small body of literature that suggests that optic nerve sheath diameter measurement may prove to be a useful tool in the emergent management of these patients. (Figure 9-1)

Background

There are a number of studies that lay the foundation for the correlation between optic nerve sheath diameter (ONSD) and ICP. The optic nerve attaches to the globe posteriorly and is sur-

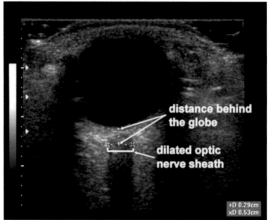

Figure 9-1 Optic Nerve Sheath. Increased intracranial pressure in the subarachnoid space results in distention of the optic nerve sheath. This is a usually most prominent 3 mm posterior to the globe. The normal optic nerve sheath measures < 5 mm in the normal adult patient. This optic nerve sheath is slightly dilated. Courtesy of Dr. Michael Blaivas.

rounded by a cerebrospinal fluid filled sheath that communicates with the intracranial cavity.

- Cadaver studies first demonstrated that increased pressure in the subarachnoid space resulted in enlargement of the bulbous portion of the nerve. Histologic studies have found that the portion of the ONS that is most distensible is that portion 3mm posterior to the globe. Thus, this has become the standard point at which ONSD is measured.
- Measurements by both sonographers and emer-

gency physicians have proven to have good interobserver reliability. Studies on normal subjects have attested to this finding.

• There is clear evidence from studies in children, that ONSDs measured by B-mode ultrasound have excellent correlation with the presence of hydrocephalus with elevated ICP.

• Upper limits of 4 mm for infants, 4.5 mm for children, and 5 mm for adults have been established from normal volunteer studies and their comparison with abnormal subjects. There is some overlap of OSND between the normal and increased ICP groups in prior studies. Kimberly et al (AEM 2/2008) reported sensitivities of 88 % and specificities of 93 % for an ONSD > 5 mm to detect ICP > 20 cm H2O in adults.

Clinical Presentation

• The various etiologies and symptoms of elevated intracranial pressure (ICP) should be familiar to all emergency physicians. The condition merits discussion in this text, as ultrasound may allow rapid bedside confirmation of the condition when suspected.

• Within the posterior orbit, the optic nerve is surrounded by a sheath containing fluid contiguous with the subarachnoid space. Increases in ICP are transmitted to the fluid within the optic nerve sheath.

• Optic nerve head edema results when the pressure of this fluid limits the flow of blood and intracellular fluid within the optic nerve itself. Direct ophthalmoscopy shows blurring of the disc margin with prominent optic cupping (papilledema), with both eyes equally affected.

Ultrasound Findings

• The optimal technique is using an axial scan (linear array probe) with the eye directed forward. Additional confirmation may be obtained by repeating the measurements in both the transverse and longitudinal (sagittal) planes. In reality, the longitudinal and transverse scans are para-axial scans as a true axial section would not directly image the nerve. The actual technique of measurement is relatively simple to teach and to perform, making it suitable for emergency physician use.

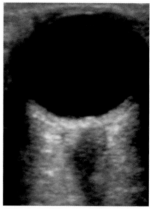

• The optic nerve sheath diameter, as measured by ultrasound, has been shown to be a sensitive indicator of elevated ICP. When measured at a point 3mm posterior to the globe, a sagittal line through the optic nerve sheath can be measured to evaluate for elevated ICP. Typically an average of 2-3 measurements on each eye are used to determine optic nerve sheath diameter

Figure 9-2 Increased Intracranial Pressure. The optic nerve sheath measures 60 millimeters in this trauma patient with elevated intracranial pressure.

• Although one cannot measure the exact ICP by ultrasound,

nerve sheath diameters greater than these accepted values are very sensitive indicators of clinically significant increased ICP's, regardless of cause. (Fig-

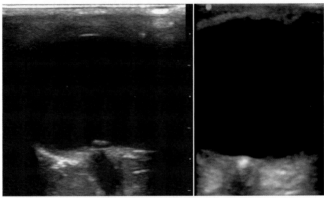

Figure 9-3 A&B Increased Intracranial Pressure with Optic Disc Edema. Differentiating papilledema from pseudopapilledema is clinically important. A) With true papilledema the optic nerve sheath is dilated. The optic nerve sheath measured 56 millimeters at a point 3 mm posterior to the globe in this patient with pseudotumor cerebri. The opening pressure on LP was > 60 cm H20 and the patient's headache improved with fluid removal. B) It should be noted that an optic nerve drusen can simulate papilledema (pseudopapilledema); however, the anechoic posterior shadowing behind the calcified nodules in the optic nerve head of a drusen will move in a distinct manner when the patient is asked to move the eye side to side. Image A courtesy of Dr. Reiner van Tonder.

ures 9-2, 9-3 A&B)

• Intracranial pressure is equally distributed throughout the cranial vault and transmission into the optic nerve sheath should affect both eyes equally. The finding of increased nerve sheath diameter in only one eye should lead the physician to pursue other possibilities for the finding (e.g. tumor obstructing fluid dynamics in that nerve sheath).

Management
 • The etiology of the increased ICP may be signaled by the patient's history or other clinical findings. Treatment should be guided according to the specific condition which precipitated the elevation in ICP.

Orbital Cellulitis
Clinical Presentation
 • Orbital cellulitis is an infection of the post-septal orbital tissues. While pre-septal infection tends to develop from skin inoculation or trauma, true orbital cellulitis is most frequently a complication of spreading sinusitis.
 • While the external appearance of both conditions may be similar, inflammation of the tissue around the extra-ocular muscles may lead to pain-limited eyeball movements in the case of orbital cellulitis. Proptosis may also be present as a distinguishing factor.
 • Visual acuity is not usually diminished until late in the disease.

Ultrasound Findings
 • Attention is given to the tissues behind the globe, and the settings on the ultrasound machine must allow for the proper depth and gain to evaluate these

areas.

• The extraocular muscles may appear thickened due to the inflammation of these tissues. Comparison with the contralateral eye may be helpful. Sub-Tenon's space may fill with fluid, resulting in a gap between the sclera and adjacent peri-orbital fat (both

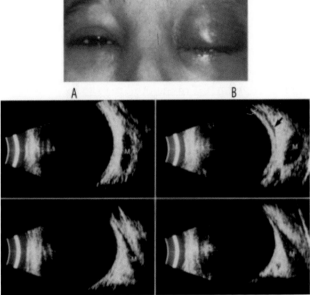

Figure 9-4 A&B Orbital Cellulitis. A) Normal right eye images demonstrating normal orbit and medial rectus muscle (M). B) Images of the left eye with orbital cellulitis demonstrating widened orbital soft tissue, thickened medial rectus muscle and fluid in the sub-Tenon's space (arrow) deep to the sclera. Orbital cellulitis results in diffuse swelling of the involved orbital structures. Reprinted with permission from Byrne S, Green R. Ultrasound of the Eye and Orbit, 2nd ed. Philadelphia, PA: Mosby; 2002.

highly echogenic). (Figure 9-4 A&B)
• The presence of multiple echolucent pockets in the orbital fat suggests an abscess with loculations. It is important to be able to recognize the difference in echogenicity of the muscle tissue from an abscess.

Management
    • While admission may not be required for pre-septal cellulitis, all cases where infection is present in the posterior orbit require admission to the hospital, IV antibiotics, and consultation with ENT, ophthalmology, or both. CT of the orbit to examine adjacent paranasal sinuses and to better define abscess cavities is recommended when there is posterior orbital involvement.

Retrobulbar hemorrhage
Clinical Presentation
    • Peri-ocular trauma may result in rupture of blood vessels posterior to the eye, but within the orbit. As this is a tightly enclosed space, hemorrhage in the retrobulbar area will initially push the globe forward. However, as the limits of anterior extrusion are reached, the condition becomes a type of compartment syndrome, with increasing retrobulbar pressure compressing nerves and blood vessels within the bony orbit. Additionally, the pressure is transmitted into the globe itself, potentially leading to the same problems seen in other forms of glaucoma.
    • With progressively worsening hemorrhage, the

patient will have marked proptosis, severe eye pain (particularly with eye movement), and varying degrees of visual disturbances.

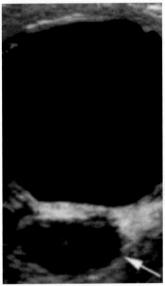

Figure 9-5 Retrobulbar Hemorrhage. Longitudinal view of the eye showing a retrobulbar hematoma represented by the hypoechoic region deep to the retina (arrow). It may be difficult to visualize a retrobulbar hemorrhage on ultrasound in some patients. This can be easy to miss if the hematoma is of similar echogenicity to surrounding structures. Reprinted with permission from Blaivas M. Bedside Emergency Department Ultrasonography in the Evaluation of Ocular Pathology. Acad Emerg Med. 2000; 7:949.

Ultrasound Findings

• Hemorrhage will be noted behind the globe. This will have the appearance of a fluid collection that may vary in echogenicity depending on the age of the hemorrhage. This may be difficult to identify on ultrasound and can be easily missed if the hemorrhage is of similar echogenicity to surrounding structures.(Figure 9-5)

Management

• Retrobulbar hemorrhage is an ophthalmologic emergency requiring intervention on the part of the emergency physician.

• A lateral canthotomy releases the pressure in the orbital cavity and should be performed once the diagnosis is made. An ophthalmologist should be consulted for definitive care.

SECTION 10: ANTERIOR CHAMBER

There are few anterior chamber findings which are assessable with 7.5 or 10 MHz linear array probes. Nevertheless, if the focus of the examination is the anterior chamber, a spacing device should be used to move the focus of interest more distal within the beam, thereby improving resolution and eliminating the contact artifact. This is of more importance when using dedicated ophthalmic probes that typically contact the eye. With linear array probes used in the ED, a closed lid and adequate gel may provide all the spacing required. Should more be desired, a glove finger filled with water and tied can provide the needed buffer.

Ultrasound Biomicroscopy

Detailed examination of the anterior chamber is possible through specialized high frequency (20-60 MHz) probes. It is termed ultrasound biomicroscopy, and has uses that are currently outside of the scope of emergency bedside scanning. With higher frequencies, and the use of a special water bath, the examiner is capable of achieving much higher resolution for evaluation of the iris, ciliary body, cornea, and angle. In addition, more precise measurements of the anterior chamber depth can be made. (Figures 10-1, 10-2)

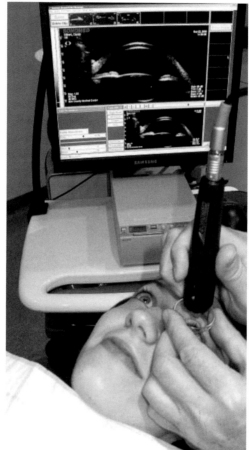

Figure 10-1 Ultrasound Biomicroscopy. This picture demonstrates the process of obtaining an image with a 35 MHz probe with a standoff bath. The image clearly displays the anterior chamber, iris, lens and ciliary body.

Pupillary Response

Assessment of pupillary response is a standard part of the examination of any head trauma patient. Abnormalities of direct or consensual responses may indicate injury to a number of different places in the neural pathways. With significant facial trauma, eyelid swelling may make it difficult to perform the examination adequately, thus ultrasound may assist in the assessment of consensual response.

Scanning technique

- The ultrasound probe must be placed at a low angle of incidence relative to the iris, allowing for maximal representation of the iris and pupil on the monitor. The probe position is a very shallow ante-

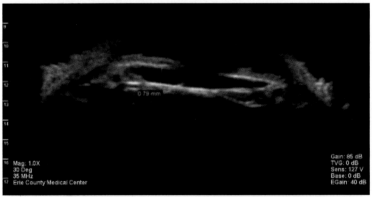

Figure 10-2 Ultrasound Biomicroscopy - Pathology. The anterior chamber can be visualized in great detail utilizing specialized high frequency probes. In this patient, a 35 MHz probe is utilized to visualize this 0.79-mm iris cyst. At this time, these probes are out of the scope of routine emergency bedside scanning but are available in many ophthalmologists' offices.

rior transverse position.
• As light is shined in the contralateral eye, the pupillary reflex can be assessed on the ultrasound image.

Management
• If an abnormal consensual response is noted, direct responses should be assessed, and the patient should be managed according to the location of the lesion.

Hyphema
As previously discussed in the trauma section, a hyphema can be easily identified on direct examination, but can also be visualized on ultrasound. Direct visualization of pathology pos-

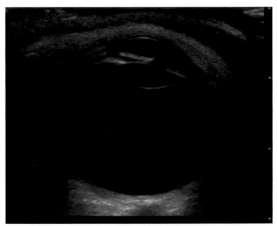

Figure 10-3 Hyphema. The echogenic area in the anterior chamber represents clotted blood in this patient with a hyphema. Courtesy of Dr. James Rippey.